HIIT

High Intensity Interval Training Guide Including Running, Cycling & Bodyweight Workouts For Weight Loss

Table of Contents

Copyright

blame be held against the publisher for any reparation, damages, or monetary loss due to the information herein, either directly or indirectly. Respective authors own all copyrights not held by the publisher.

The information herein is offered for informational purposes solely, and is universal as so. The presentation of the information is without contract or any type of guarantee assurance.

The trademarks that are used are without any consent, and the publication of the trademark is without permission or backing by the trademark owner. All trademarks and brands within this book are for clarifying purposes only and are the owned by the owners themselves, not affiliated with this document.

Introduction

Whether you are looking at losing weight, improving your running speed, boosting your general body fitness or gaining those six packs you have been yearning for, HIIT bike training won't let you down. According to a study conducted by the American College of Sports Medicine, HIIT was the most preferred cardio exercise in 2014.

This book will teach you everything there is to know about HIIT bike training. In this book, you will learn the basics of HIIT and how to harness its power in getting faster, stronger, fitter and even lose weight with much ease among many other health benefits.

An Overview of HIIT

HIIT (High-Intensity Interval Training) is a cardio exercise developed many years ago by track coaches to help them prepare athletes. As we are aware, a cardio exercise is any exercise that has the effect of increasing your heart rate. That is exactly what HIIT does to your body. Initially, HIIT was known as 'speed play', which describes the very nature of HIIT, as we shall see as we progress with our discussion. So, what exactly is HIIT? Let's learn that next.

What is HIIT?

In HIIT training, you put 100% of your effort through intense quick bursts of exercise followed by short recovery periods, which at times can as well be active. In simple terms, it means that you will be cycling or running or whichever way you do your cardio exercise very fast briefly and then follow it with low-intensity exercise such as walking or complete rest. In other words, HIIT entails taking intervals of high-intensity exercise such sprinting or cycling and then following it with intervals of low-intensity exercises such as walking or completely taking a rest. Sounds familiar now, doesn't it? Well, here is how you stand to gain when you engage in HIIT:

- A well-done HIIT increases your metabolic rate. According to Eric Salvador, HIIT leads to excess post-exercise consumption of oxygen. This means that your body will increase its metabolic rate to supply this oxygen. Salvador says that this can continue up to a period of 48 hours, which simply means that you continue burning fat hours after a single HIIT.

- HIIT is very quick and convenient. Your daily schedules no longer need to be the excuse for that protruding belly which is due to excess fat. With 30 minutes or less, HIIT would have achieved its goals. Very convenient in that you can do it anywhere be it in an hotel, in a park, gym or anywhere.

- You don't need any equipment to do HIIT. Additionally, you do not need to go shopping for gym. These exercises entail use of your body weight given that their focus is to get your heart rate up and keep it high. The end result is optimal muscle building and retention combined with fat loss and enhanced calorie burning. It is a cheap exercise with profound results.

- Efficiency: HIIT has been proven to burn more fat in 15 minute sessions done 3 times a week than running on a treadmill for an hour.

- HIIT helps preserve muscle mass given that it is an anaerobic activity. This makes it ideal for developing abs or six-pack without shedding body fat.

- It triggers increased production of the human growth hormone (HGH), which means that you will burn more fat and preserve more muscle mass.

- The fact that the exercise mimics real life situations whereby you engage in short bursts of activity makes it a great routine.

- The exercise is ideal in toning and shaping the lower body.

Our bodies were made to move and as such, we have to move them. That said, to keep our body muscles in shape, then we must move them. This movement makes them stronger and a strong muscle is responsible for a more efficient and healthy body. Your heart is muscle in itself. A cardio exercise therefore makes it stronger and more efficient in performing its roles key among them supplying oxygen to body cells. This enables your cells to burn more fat hence eliminating excess fats in the body; your body needs oxygen for metabolism processes to take place so when there is more oxygen, you get to burn more fats. That is how much you need a cardio exercise! Let's discuss some possible ways through which you stand to gain from exercising irrespective of the nature of exercise you are engaging in.

General benefits of doing an exercise

Before we get started, it is perhaps important that you appreciate the fact that regular exercises are critical for a healthy body and mind. In any case, too much work without play will surely make Jack a dull boy! So, why is it that you should exercise? Let's look at these in greater detail.

Exercise will help you control your weight

As we all know, exercise helps you burn more calories, which means that the more the intensity of exercise, the more calories you burn. This pushes your body into a calorie deficit condition, making it to start burning stored fat, which in turn means that you will start losing weight.

Better mood

Exercise prompts the brain and other body parts to produce feel good hormones (endorphins) making you to be in a better mood. The endorphins are known to produce a positive feeling that is similar to that of morphine (you feel euphoric or runner's high). Endorphins are also known to help reduce the perception of pain and act as sedatives. You also get to feel more confident and with greater self-esteem when you exercise.

Regular exercises will boost your energy levels

Exercise will give you stronger muscles; stronger muscles can endure strain. When you exercise regularly, you push your body to up its energy production in order to meet your increased energy demands. When you exercise, your body increases muscle mass, reduces body fat, increases the heart's pumping volume, improves circulation, lowers fat in the blood like bad cholesterol, enhances the body's blood sugar regulation and enhances mood and mental capacity. All these work together to enhance your energy levels. Additionally, physical activities supply oxygen and nutrients to the tissues, which in turn boosts your cardiovascular system.

Exercises can help you prevent or manage a wide range of health issues

Physical activity helps in keeping such health problems like heart diseases, cancer, high blood pressure, depression, cardiovascular diseases and many others at bay. It also helps prevent bone loss, manage blood pressure, manage stress, fight anxiety and depression, manage blood cholesterol and many others. Interestingly, it also helps in fighting addictions and in sharpening memory.

Exercise boosts the quality of your sleep

Physical activity can help you fall asleep faster and sleep soundly. However, don't exercise just before bedtime otherwise your body is too active to fall asleep!

Exercises also boost your sex life

It reduces the chances of erectile dysfunction in men and enhances arousal for women.

This list of benefits is definitely not conclusive; each type of exercise has its unique benefits besides the ones listed here. For instance, HIIT bike training can help you boost speed if you are training for a competition and even help you get fitter. Even if you want to make your muscles stronger, or lose more fat, HIIT bike training is a good starting point. If you need to lose more fat, do not worry, let me now take you through several HIIT workouts that will help you achieve your goals.

HIIT Workouts

In this chapter, my aim is to open up your mind to the several options that you have if you are interested in trying HIIT. We will therefore describe these workouts precisely and then move on to HIIT bike training, which is the core of the subsequent chapters of this book.

Sprinting

Sprinting has been found to be an effective way of going about your high intensity interval training. It involves intervals of high speed running followed by short periods of walking or taking complete rests. I usually do not recommend for people who are still not in shape this workout as they risk being injured. Even for those who are sure about their physical fitness, there are rules to be adhered to in this workout.

It starts by you heading to a track and letting yourself all-out. Start by warming up and then take your 20 seconds sprint. Follow it immediately with say 10 seconds jump and then take a 30 seconds rest or walk. This exercise has been found to be very effective in burning calories.

Push-Ups

Push-ups are ideal for building your muscles and making them stronger. With this exercise, you have to do at least 30 pushups or press-ups without taking a rest. This is then followed by low-intensity training that allows your body to recover; you can follow this with complete rest. Here is how to go about it:

1. Get into plank position with your hands on the ground when they are directly under your shoulders; your legs should be about hip width apart.

2. Bend the elbows and the entire body until you touch the ground while you keep your elbows tucked against the sides and while your body is positioned in a straight line. Move down as far as possible then return to the start position then repeat the exercise 30 times.

Jump squats

In this exercise, you squat and then take a small jump forward and back to your squat position. Repeat the exercise for at least 45 times and then immediately follow it with a low intensity exercise to allow your body to recover. If you like this exercise, use it consistently since it has some post effects on your muscles that can turn into pain if not continuously used.

Sit-ups

1. To do this start by laying on your back having your knees bent as your feet are on the floor then tighten the core then pull your head using your abs and then back off the ground until you are actually sitting upright while your back is perpendicular to the floor.

2. Lie back slowly as you pull your abs and then get to the start position and finally repeat the exercise 50 times.

Tricep Dip

Start by getting onto all fours while you face the ceiling with your knees bent at 90 degrees right above your toes while your hands are on the ground right under your shoulders. At this time, your fingers should be facing forward while your back is straight such that your core is now parallel to the ground.

Bend your elbows while they are tucked in so that you lower your butt as close to the ground as you possibly can. You can now push back up then repeat the exercise for 10 times.

Other HIIT workouts that you could try include split jumps, jump squats, and burpees just to mention a few. Although there are many other workouts for HIIT, the ultimate aim is to ensure that you continue burning fat hours after the exercise. To attain this with greater ease, it is perhaps best to try using HIIT bike training to burn even more calories and achieve all the benefits that come with HIIT. We will discuss HIIT bike training in the subsequent chapters.

HIIT Bike Training

In the previous chapter, we looked at some possible workouts that you can use for high intensity interval training. I deliberately left out cycling because we dedicate this book to learning how to do it successfully. Many professionals recommend cycling for those who want to increase their speed on the track, lose weight, and strengthen their muscles just to mention a few of the ways through which you stand to gain when you do HIIT bike training.

Why HIIT bike training?

Many studies give bike training authenticity as the number one way of getting the best from HIIT. Here is why you should try HIIT training.

The fats factor

One undisputable fact is that bike riding burns more calories than many other exercises. Additionally, you also continue burning calories even at rest. When you push your body to increase metabolism, it responds by burning stored fat in order to meet energy demands. Obviously, your diet should be low in calories to ensure that the body can easily get into a state of calorie deficit so that it can burn stored fat for energy.

Since your goal is to push the body to burn stored fat, you should aim at doing high intensity riding (I will show you how later on in this book).

Also, bike training increases your lactate threshold (*that point at which your legs start to sting like a bee bite and you are left with no option except to slow down*) hence making you a high calorie consumer. This means that you will be burning a lot more calories even after the exercise.

The speed factor

High intensity riding raises your VOX2Max and lactate threshold. A high intensity riding increases your volume of oxygen consumption to maximum (VOX2Max). When you become a high oxygen consumer, you develop a robust cardiovascular system that ensures enough supply of oxygen-rich blood. This ensures good coordination between your muscles and the nervous system, which in turn boosts your speed and muscles endurance.

Lactate threshold denotes that point at which you legs start to sting like a bee bite and you are left with no option except to slow down. Intervals increase your lactate threshold so you transform into a faster rider with high endurance.

The energy factor

Energy comes when we have a healthy body that is adequately supplied with blood and oxygen coupled with good nervous coordination. This is what bike riding is all about. Our muscles also become stronger as we continue to add more strain onto them. So, if you are a habitual cyclist, you will not need to do a different session to strengthen your muscles.

So, now that you have understood what HIIT bike cycling is all about, let's now narrow everything down to discussing about the specific HIIT bike cycling techniques that you should be using.

An indoor cycling jumps

This exercise can be performed indoors or out on the roads. With your hands steady on the handlebars, move your body from the hips back and forward over the seat of your bicycle then in an upright position. Once you have achieved this position, hold a jump at each position.

The swaying motion combined with the efforts that you are using to balance and hold the bike grip produces an amazing tone on your muscles. Dr. Tabata says that you can integrate this training with your music beats. How?

He says that you can choose to go for sets of say 10 of these exercises. You will then let the music beats dictate your motion forth and forward as you do the jump workouts. This he says will then kill the boredom. Since it is high intensity interval training, you should allow yourself a 1 minute rest after performing say 10 sets of jumps. This allows your muscles to recover.

You can also interchange sets of seated and standing jumps to gain maximum fat burnouts. Always strive to gain maximum control of your bike by increasing resistance. Bike jumps are ideal for producing maximum effects on your muscles and has an effect of strengthening them. It is also a good way to burn calories.

Interval hill sprints

Just like normal sprints towards the hills, resistance is also higher when you climb a hill while riding than when riding on a flat surface. It tests the power of your legs.

When doing this bike exercise, first lower resistance and let your leg do as many revolutions per minute as it is possible. Carefully come out of your seat at intervals of 5 seconds to engage your body wholly to the exercise. Ensure that your hips are in uniform motion with your legs as well. The idea is to make all the muscular parts of the body participate in the exercise to enable maximum calorie burnout.

Use the first ten seconds of beginning this exercise to gain your momentum and the next ten seconds to maintain this momentum. After each sprint, allow yourself 1 to 2 minutes rest though an easy cycling perhaps on a flat surface is quite perfect.

However, if you are doing this exercise for the first time, do not make it so vigorous; start it moderately and gradually increase your speed until when you are fit enough to do it like pros do it.

Tabata cycling

Dr. Tabata came out with one of what has been considered the most effective cardio exercise among many professionals given that it produces much more profound results than normal aerobic exercises.

This involves 20 seconds workouts and 10 seconds rest. During the 20 seconds, Tabata advises that you sprint i.e. cycle, at least to a speed of 80 to 90 percent of your maximum speed. The 20 seconds should therefore be your maximum intensity workout interval. After the 20 seconds, slow to at least 60 percent of your maximum speed to allow recovery.

Strive to achieve at least 8 or 12 repeated Tabata cycling and burn fats faster than usual! This Tabata style of HIIT workout has gained popularity as the most preferred high interval intensity training. It is also perhaps one of the most intense workouts. It is very effective for strengthening muscles, gaining body fitness and losing fats. Amazingly, it is the shortest workout.

Do your 8-12 intervals and go on with your other activities. The effects will last for many hours.

Hovering over your seat

With your hands firmly on the handlebars, move your hips back and have your butt literally hovering above your seat at say 3 inches. Hold on to this position for 45 seconds. Repeat this exercise for 1 to 3 intervals in addition to your daily workout routine. If you can do it while riding at the same time, perfect.

There are those who have no idea how to use their hamstrings when doing a workout like bicycle riding. This workout is your best if you are such a person. This gives high intense sensation to your hamstrings and quads. Ensure that you do not hold too tightly the handlebars. Just give it a light touch but giving you control over your bike.

I hope you have learnt about other workouts that you did not know about HIIT bike training program. In the next chapter, let us shift focus into learning about preparations for this workout.

Training Plans for Cyclists

Recently I was part of a session when one of the attendees challenged me to provide them with a sample plan they can use for their HIIT bike training program. Well, he got me off guard, so I promised him that I will put it down in this tutorial.

As you have been learning about HIIT, I know that you now understand that the harder you ride, the better you get at it. Well, this is easier said than done especially when you don't have a plan. As such, a workout plan can make the difference between success and failure in HIIT. In simple terms, plan your ride and get better at it. If you want to become a better rider then you cannot just woke up and starting riding at random.

Planning your workouts requires that you understand how energy is used in each activity. We will discuss the contribution of various energy systems to any exercise (these are dependent on the duration within which the exercise takes). The body's use of energy can be described in three energy systems: aerobic, glycolytic and ATP systems. How much each system is used is however dependent on the duration and intensity of each activity:

1. ATP is the one responsible for on the spot energy. It uses adenosine triphosphate (ATP) to produce this energy. It is the sprinter in us. It only produces this energy for a few glorious seconds by breaking the ATP chemically to supply a quick surge of energy. ATP energy will only last you 10 to 30 seconds. Once this energy is gone, you have to give your body time to replenish its stores of ATP. That is where recovery time in your workouts comes in.

2. The glycolytic system also referred to as the anaerobic system lasts much longer than the ATP system. It is however, not so intense. You can work your muscles for 2 to 10 minutes in an anaerobic system. The system breaks down glycogen to lactic acid to rejuvenate an oxygen-deprived muscle. It is the energy that sustains you after that sprint or hill climb.

3. The other system is the aerobic system. It is responsible for the power behind that long riding on the mountain. In this system, blood supplies oxygen to the body muscles. This oxygen is then used to break down glycogen into carbon dioxide. This provides a sustainable energy for your pedals. Aerobic system is the power behind those long rides exceeding 5 minutes or so.

With HIIT bike routines, the ultimate goal is to train the aerobic system so that it can last much longer. So, how do we it? Here is how:

Step 1: Start by strength enhancement

Muscles are usually the weak links for any rider. It is not that these muscles are usually weak but because they give out too quickly. Once a feeling of exhaustion stems from your leg muscles, then your workout plan is finished no matter what. To curb this problem, I recommend that that you aim for about 60% of your maximum for say 2 weeks depending on the period within which you want to train. This should continue until your muscles are fully accustomed to strain. This step is crucial because the muscles unlike the lungs and the heart do not recover that fast. This low intensity cycling is therefore quite useful.

Step 2: Transition to stronger cycling

Once you have made your muscles stronger, it is time you move on to more intense training. This step starts by you reaching your aerobic threshold. The aerobic threshold is the point when your body starts going to an oxygen debt although you can still maintain this state for at least 30 minutes if the situation dictates. If you can maintain this position for over 30 minutes, then you are not trying as hard as I expect it to be. If you cannot maintain it for over 15 minutes, then kudos; you are doing a good job!

It is important that you are able to identify your threshold point. You can easily find out that point by taking a hill sprint with your bike taking note of your revolutions per minute (rpm) until you hear your breathing pattern change.

The key to making this stage effective for your early HIIT bike training plan is ensuring that there is enough tension on your muscles during the entire period. Keeping a steady pedal stroke with a still upper body is also another secret.

This stage should be done in at least 2 or 3 intervals per workout followed by a 10 minutes recovery period.

Step 3: Breaking down the pedal stroke

This stage should be at the peak of your training; I advise that you use the top gear. This will help you accelerate, stand on your bike and hold on to the rolling bike until you reach the end without having to switch gears.

Do a smooth acceleration settling back to the saddle while ensuring that you do not miss any pedal stroke. You can decide to use a starting point and a stopping end that allows 30 seconds of recovery period in between.

Since this stage is advanced, 6 intervals for each workout is sufficient. A recovery period of 5 minutes is okay.

Step 4: High spin

You can perform this in an easy or your comfortable gear. It therefore does not require that you go uphill or any raised surface. A flat surface will do fine.

If you are a beginner (of course form matters so much), start at a 100rpm and accelerate to at least 130 revolutions per minute. You should not be worried if your heart rate reaches the aerobic threshold so fast. Since you have been working on strengthening your body in the last stages, it will easily adapt to this change.

I really do not want your speed to peak before the maximum so we will limit this phase for 10 minutes followed by a recovery. Since this is quite easy to do, you can do it during your recovery hours or days.

Although you now have the basic workout stages that you need to observe, it might probably be inadequate if I fail to prepare you for this noble exercise. Each workout should always start with a 20 minutes warm up though I advise that if you have more time at your disposal, you can do 30 to 40 minutes warm up to prepare you for the task. It should not be a challenge if you are psychologically prepared for the challenge.

The other thing to observe is that you should never ignore recovery time. Do not let your training partners strain you more than necessary. Recovery period as important as the training itself.

Rest makes it easy to adapt to the exercise Resting also helps the body to renew capabilities and systems allowing you to be better prepared for the next activity.

Rest and recovery are very helpful in restoring energy and repairing muscles and tissues allowing you to perform better in the next exercise since you can adapt your body to the system of that activity.

Enhances aerobic endurance. When you rest or go through recovery, you enhance aerobic endurance or your capacity to have sufficient oxygen support so that you can withstand difficult and tiring physical activity.

In a nutshell, when you engage in higher intensity periods, you push your body to create a metabolic demand, which helps in long term fat loss and overall conditioning while any rests (low intensity period) in between helps you to recover and even use the aerobic energy system.

Note:

You do not need to have this workout interfere with your daily schedules. You can still ride for faster for short bursts but still burn large amount of calories in your body. So your plan needs not to conform to the others that you will read about in the various websites you come across. Just look at the time you have at your disposal and schedule your time in light of your personal commitments. Here is why recovery time is crucial in your HIIT bike training routines.

Note: Different cyclists use different plans to achieve their goals. However, these plans are not quite different in their principles.

You could easily assume that HIIT bike training is just a single exercise that magically makes you achieve all the benefits. However, it actually isn't; you have to engage in several forms of HIIT bike training if you are to achieve the different benefits that come with HIIT bike training. Let's have a look at these in the next chapter.

HIIT Bike Training Programs

In the previous sections, we assumed that the approach is the same in each training session whether training for fitness, speed enhancement or fat loss. Well, this was a wrong assumption although it was meant to explain what we were discussing at that time. There are various disciplines when it comes to bike training and it is important that you understand which discipline fits each situation. Each of these disciplines will call for a different training program. In this section, we shift focus to some of these disciplines.

Road racing

This group of cyclists are said to possess a lot of endurance. Several studies have shown that aerobic power is quite high in this group of cyclists. Most of the people who use this program are athletes who wish to boost their speed.

A measurement called lactate threshold is majorly used in this program to measure performance. Lactate threshold is the point at which your legs start to sting forcing you to slow down. Interval training is said to increase you lactate threshold hence making you a high calorie consumer. It therefore means that lactate threshold measures your speed as well as fat loss rate. Professional athletes who have high lactate threshold can become faster riders, burn more calories and enhance their general body fitness.

Road racing is therefore ideal for those aiming to improve their speed, lose fats, get fit among other general health concerns.

Track racing

Track racing is another bike training program. If you want to run fast, then you have to really run fast; that is what track racing is all about. Track racing is low intensity interval training but it can really boost your speed and fitness.

It involves you setting off for a long distance riding slotting in intervals coupled with recovery periods. Researchers at MacMaster University found out that this is good for recovery periods especially for those who have been doing high intensity training and want to take a rest.

It has an effect of strengthening your cardiovascular system; a stronger cardio system sufficiently supplies the body with oxygen-rich blood. Muscles get better at using that oxygenated blood. The coordination between your nervous system and the muscles get super charged and the result is increased revolutions per minute. Your speed is improved as well.

While on the track, begin with say a 300 meters at 80 percent of your maximum speed. Include a 2 or 3 minutes recovery time where you can choose to go slow or take complete rest. Increase these distances ensuring that you take recovery periods nicely. Once you become a pro, you should start with great distances.

Mountain Biking

This involves cycling off the road mostly over rough hilly terrain. Some prefer using specially designed bikes for this exercise. Unlike the two programs we have discussed earlier, mountain biking is a very high intensity training routine.

The good news with this program is that you really do need to spend a lot of time; 10 minutes is probably enough to push you to the edge!

Mountain biking has been proven to be a very fast and an effective way of getting faster. It raises your VOX2Max i.e. it raises your oxygen consumption to maximum level. You have probably heard some people say that those who live in hilly landscapes make good athletes. Well, nothing can be further from that truth. Raised VOX2Max greatly improves your speed and energy level.

Mountain biking starts with identifying your favorite trail. You should set up the sprints at certain sections of the trail and areas that are a bit flat as recovery sections of the exercise. Repeat the hill climbs as intervals for maximum results. Make your training long enough and intense to test your skills and endurance.

Stationary bike training

Stationery bikes are easy ways of training. The advantage with them is that you can probably watch TV while you engage in your training sessions. Nonetheless, you need a lot of discipline for this to work. I advise that you set goals that you would wish to achieve from the workout in advance.

Do some off-the-saddle hill climbing incorporating high resistance, low revolutions per minute and standing on the pedals. This would produce effects on your hamstrings and muscles. Shift to some sprints with lower resistance but keeping your revolutions per minute as high as it is possible. Some cruising will require that you go for moderate resistance and slower revolutions.

If you can do at least a 30 minutes workout each day of the week, this is definitely a plus for you. I know of some great athletes who do it for over 2 hours. However, do not add extra time to daily workouts suddenly. The increase in training duration should be gradual to avoid possible injuries. If you want to recover, try to incorporate easy rides in your stationery bike to allow your body to recover.

Conclusion

I hope you have learnt something or many things you did not know about HIIT bike training. Although the subject seems to be complex, you definitely stand to gain when you engage in regular HIIT bike training routines regularly. In summary, if you want to:

1. **Get lean muscle:** You should do HIIT 3-4 times weekly depending on your ability to recover.

2. **Gain strength:** Do HIIT at most once a week ensuring that you have attained full recovery before lifting again.

3. **Put on some muscle:** Do HIIT one or two times in a week.

4. **Enhance endurance i.e. long distance or sprint distance:** HIIT might not be what you are looking for if your goal is to run marathon or engage in a triathlon. However, you can use HIIT if you want to go for several rounds in a fight.

Bonus Content

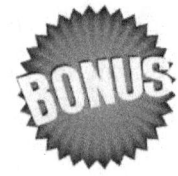

As a token of our appreciation Grand Reveur Publications would like to give you access to our exclusive bonus content (including free eBooks!).

Exclusive pre-release access to our latest eBooks Free Grand Reveur eBooks during promotional periods.

A method ANYONE can use to publish their own book and make passive income

To receive this bonus content visit the following web site:

https://ignorelimits.leadpages.net/grandreveur publications/

As this is a limited time offer it would be a shame to miss out, I recommend grabbing these bonuses before reading on.